SECOND EDITION

EKG

In a Heartbeat

Karen M. **Ellis**, RN

Touro Infirmary, New Orleans

D0223805

Pearson

Boston   Columbus   Indianapolis   New York   San Francisco
Upper Saddle River   Amsterdam   Cape Town   Dubai   London
Madrid   Milan   Munich   Paris   Montreal   Toronto   Delhi   Mexico City
Sao Paulo   Sydney   Hong Kong   Seoul   Singapore   Taipei   Tokyo

Library of Congress Cataloging-in-Publication Data

Ellis, Karen M., author.
   EKG in a heartbeat / Karen M. Ellis. — 2nd ed.
      p. ; cm.
   Includes index.
   ISBN-13: 978-0-13-249932-3
   ISBN-10: 0-13-249932-0
   1. Electrocardiography—Handbooks, manuals, etc. I. Title.
   [DNLM: 1. Electrocardiography—Handbooks. WG 39]
   RC683.5.E5E44 2011
   616.1'207547—dc22

                              2010046408

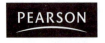

www.pearsonhighered.com

10 9 8 7 6 5 4 3

ISBN 0-13-249932-0
ISBN 978-0-13-249932-3

Publisher: Julie Levin Alexander
Executive Assistant & Supervisor: Regina Bruno
Editor-in-Chief: Mark Cohen
Executive Editor: Joan Gill
Development Editor: Melissa Kerian
Associate Editor: Bronwen Glowacki
Editorial Assistant: Mary Ellen Ruitenberg
Director of Marketing: David Gesell
Executive Marketing Manager: Katrin Beacom
Marketing Specialist: Michael Sirinides
Managing Production Editor: Patrick Walsh
Production Liaison: Patricia Gutierrez
Composition: Laserwords Private Limited
Production Editor: Erika Jordan/Rebecca Lazure
Manufacturing Manager: Alan Fischer
Creative Director: Christy Mahon
Art Director: Kristine Carney
Printer/Binder: Edwards Brothers Malloy
Cover Printer: Edwards Brothers Malloy

Contents

12-Lead EKG Interpretation

Acknowledgments

To my husband Lee for always being there with love and support—and for rescuing me from computer-induced fits of frustration.

To my editors Melissa Kerian and Mark Cohen for guiding me through this process and being supportive of this effort.

Introduction

You're busy. And you've got a mountain of information to master as part of your position (or desired position) in healthcare. So you could really use a quick reference on EKG interpretation. You need a pocket guide.

But which one? There are lots of them out there.

Unlike some pocket guides, which are miniature versions of textbooks a few hundred pages long, this pocket guide has the tools you need to help you read rhythm strips and 12-lead EKGs, **but it doesn't take hundreds of pages to say it.** Fast, accurate, and to the point. When you're standing at a patient's bedside you need a memory-jogger, not a treatise on EKG.

But a word of caution. This is not intended as an elementary text on electrocardiography. It's a "how to do it" kind of book. It presumes at least a basic knowledge of EKG principles. If you want a comprehensive EKG textbook, consider my textbook *EKG Plain and Simple.*

Contained within this pocket guide are the tools for rhythm and 12-lead EKG interpretation: how to calculate heart rate, how to determine intervals, how to analyze a rhythm strip, rhythm interpretation words of wisdom, pictorials for rhythm interpretation and MI localization, as well as info on axis, hypertrophy, bundle branch blocks and hemiblocks. There are checklists, algorithms, tables, EKGs, rhythm strips, and more.

So when you need EKG info **right now,** just reach into your pocket. *EKG in a Heartbeat* is the perfect fit–for your pocket and your needs.

Hope you find it helpful.

Sincerely,

Karen Ellis

Basic Rhythm Interpretation

How to Analyze a Rhythm Strip

Rhythm Interpretation Words of Wisdom

- All matching upright P waves in Lead II are sinus P waves until proven otherwise.

- Sinus rhythms must have an atrial rate less than or equal to 160 **in a supine resting adult.**

- All wide-QRS beats without preceding P waves are ventricular until proven otherwise.

- If the QRS complexes look alike, the T waves that follow them should also look alike. A T wave that suddenly changes shape when the QRS complexes don't is hiding a P wave inside it.

- The most common cause of an unexplained pause is a nonconducted PAC.

- Absence of conduction does not necessarily imply a block. Block implies a pathologic process. Absence of conduction may be simply due to refractoriness, a normal physiologic process.

5 Steps to Rhythm Interpretation

1. Are there QRS complexes?
   - If there are no QRS complexes, the rhythm is either asystole, P wave asystole, or ventricular fibrillation. All other rhythms have QRS complexes.
   - If there are QRSs, are they the same shape, or does the shape vary?
   - If there are no QRSs, skip to question 4.

How to Analyze a Rhythm Strip (cont'd)

2. Is the rhythm regular, regular but interrupted, or irregular?
   - Compare the R-R intervals (the distance between consecutive QRSs).

3. What is the heart rate?
   - If the heart rate is >100, the patient has a **tachycardia.**
   - If the heart rate is <60, the patient has a **bradycardia.**

4. Are there P waves?
   - If so, what is their relationship to the QRS? In other words, are the Ps always in the same place relative to the QRS, or are the Ps in different places with each beat?
   - Are any Ps not followed by a QRS?
   - Are the Ps all the same shape, or does the shape vary?
   - Is the P-P interval regular?

5. What are the PR, QRS, and QT intervals?
   - Are the intervals within normal limits, or are they too short or too long?
   - Are the intervals constant, or do they vary?

How to Determine the Regularity of a Rhythm

There are three types of regularity:

1. **Regular.** R-R intervals are constant and vary only by one or two little blocks. On the following strip, the R-R intervals are all about 20 little blocks apart. The rhythm is regular.

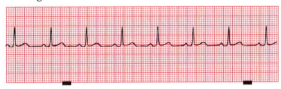

2. **Regular but interrupted.** This is a regular rhythm interrupted by premature beats or pauses. Strip A shows a regular rhythm interrupted by a premature beat (indicated by the dot) and the short pause that normally follows it. Strip B shows a regular rhythm interrupted by a pause.

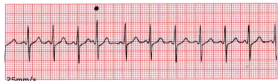

A 25mm/s

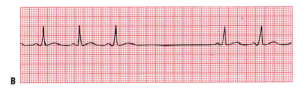

B

How to Determine the Regularity of a Rhythm (cont'd)

3. **Irregular.** R-R intervals vary throughout the strip.

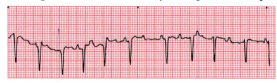

How to Calculate Heart Rate (Methods)

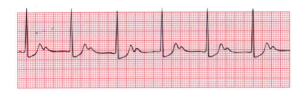

1. Memorize this sequence of numbers: 300-150-100-75-60-50-43-37-33-30. This represents the number of big blocks between consecutive QRS complexes divided into 300. On the strip the QRSs are all five big blocks apart. Go to the 5th number in our sequence–the heart rate is 60.

2. Count the number of little blocks between consecutive QRSs and divide into 1,500. On the strip the QRSs are all 25 little blocks apart. $1,500 \div 25 = 60$.

3. Count the number of QRSs on a 6-secs strip and multiply by 10. There are six QRS complexes on this 6-secs strip, so the **mean** (**average**) **heart rate** is 60. This is the least accurate method.

Regularity-Based Heart Rate Calculation

Rhythm Regularity	Kind of Heart Rate to Calculate
Regular	One heart rate, using big or little block method
Regular but interrupted by premature beats	One heart rate (ignoring premature beats)
Regular but interrupted by pauses	Range slowest to fastest, plus mean rate
Irregular	Range slowest to fastest, plus mean rate

How to Calculate Heart Rate (Chart)

Count the number of little blocks between QRS complexes and follow the dots to the HR.

Blocks	HR	Blocks	HR	Blocks	HR
1	1,500	21	71	41	37
2	750	22	68	42	36
3	500	23	65	43	35
4	375	24	62	44	34
5	300	25	60	45	33
6	250	26	58	46	33
7	214	27	56	47	32
8	187	28	54	48	31
9	167	29	52	49	31
10	150	30	50	50	30
11	137	31	48	51	29
12	125	32	47	52	29
13	115	33	45	53	28
14	107	34	44	54	28
15	100	35	43	55	27
16	94	36	42	56	27
17	88	37	41	57	26
18	83	38	39	58	26
19	79	39	38	59	25
20	75	40	37	60	25

How to Determine Intervals

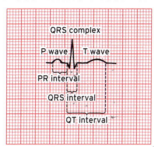

PR Interval

Count the number of little blocks between the beginning of the P wave and the beginning of the QRS complex. Multiply by 0.04 secs. Normal PR interval is 0.12 to 0.20 secs (between three and five little blocks).

QRS Interval

Count the number of little blocks between the beginning and end of the QRS complex. Multiply by 0.04 secs. Normal QRS interval is <0.12 secs (less than three little blocks wide).

QT Interval

Count the number of little blocks between the beginning of the QRS complex and the end of the T wave. Multiply by 0.04 secs. Normal QT interval varies with the heart rate. At heart rates between 60 and 100, the QT interval should be less than half the R-R interval.

How to Identify Sinus Rhythms

The sinus node is the acknowledged king of the conduction system's pacemaker cells. And there are only two ways for the sinus node king to relinquish its throne:

1. By illness or death of the sinus node, requiring someone to step in for it (escape)
2. By being overthrown by a lower pacemaker (usurpation/ irritability)

Though they can be irregular at times, sinus rhythms are for the most part regular. They're like the ticking of a clock—predictable and expected. The inherent rate of the sinus node is 60 to 100, but this rate can go higher or lower if the sinus node is acted on by the sympathetic or parasympathetic nervous system. The patient's tolerance of these rhythms will depend in large part on the heart rate. Heart rates that are too fast or too slow can cause symptoms of decreased cardiac output.

Treatment is not needed unless symptoms develop. At that time, the goal is to return the heart rate to normal.

Sinus rhythms are the standard against which all other rhythms are compared. Here are the criteria for sinus rhythms:

- **Upright matching P waves in Lead II followed by a QRS (P may be inverted in V_1)** *and*
- **PR intervals constant** *and*
- **QRS interval $<$0.12 secs** *and*
- **Heart rate $\leq$160 in a supine resting adult**

Sinus Rhythms Pictorial

Sinus Rhythm (SR)

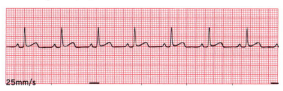

25mm/s

Criteria: Matching upright P waves in Lead II followed by a QRS, constant PR interval between 0.12 and 0.20 secs, QRS interval <0.12 secs, HR 60 to 100.
Cause: Normal.
Adverse Effects: None.
Treatment: None.

Sinus Bradycardia (SB)

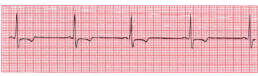

Criteria: Same as sinus rhythm, except HR <60.
Cause: Vagal stimulation, MI, hypoxia, medications, well-conditioned athlete.
Adverse Effects: Signs of decreased cardiac output (dizziness, weakness, diaphoresis, hypotension, syncope)–or no symptoms at all.
Treatment: Oxygen, atropine if symptomatic. Often no treatment needed.

Sinus Rhythms Pictorial (cont'd)

Sinus Tachycardia (ST)

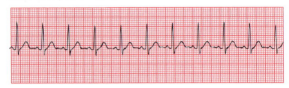

Criteria: Same as sinus rhythm, except HR >100 (and ≤160 in a supine resting adult).

Cause: Medications (atropine, bronchodilators, etc.), emotional upset, fever, pulmonary embolus, congestive heart failure, MI, hypoxia, blood loss.

Adverse Effects: Often well-tolerated but can cause signs of decreased cardiac output if HR too fast; increases the stress on the heart–can lead to heart failure after acute MI.

Treatment: Treat the cause.

Sinus Arrhythmia (SA)

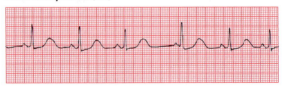

Criteria: Same as sinus rhythm, except the **rhythm is irregular**–the longest R-R interval exceeds the shortest by four little blocks or more.

Cause: Breathing pattern; rarely heart disease.

Adverse Effects: Usually none.

Treatment: Usually none required.

Sinus Rhythms Pictorial (cont'd)

Sinus Arrest

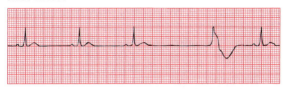

Criteria: A pause that interrupts a sinus rhythm. The pause is not a multiple of the previous R-R intervals.
Cause: Sinus node ischemia, digitalis toxicity, hypoxia, vagal stimulation.
Adverse Effects: Usually none, though long pauses can cause signs of decreased cardiac output.
Treatment: Usually none needed. Atropine if symptomatic.

Sinus Exit Block

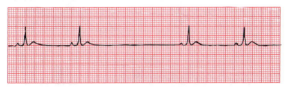

Criteria: A pause that interrupts a sinus rhythm. The pause **is** a multiple of the previous R-R intervals.
Cause, adverse effects, treatment: Same as sinus arrest.

How to Identify Atrial Rhythms

Though the atrium is not considered an inherent pacemaker like the sinus node, AV junction, and ventricle (it rarely functions in an escape role), the atrium is indeed another pacemaker of the heart. It is best known for usurping the underlying sinus rhythm and stealing control away, resulting in very rapid heart rates that can leave the patients symptomatic. Every now and then the atrium will fire more slowly and produce rhythms with heart rates less than 100.

Treatment is aimed at converting the rhythm back to sinus rhythm, or, if that is not possible, returning the heart rate to more normal levels.

Atrial rhythms vary in their presentation. Some rhythms have obvious P waves. Others have no Ps at all–instead, they have fibrillatory or flutter waves between the QRS complexes. Some atrial rhythms are regular and others are completely irregular, even chaotic. Though most atrial rhythms are rapid, a few are slower.

Unlike sinus rhythms, which have a common set of criteria, atrial rhythms have multiple and variable possible criteria. If the rhythm or beat in question meets *any* of these criteria, it is atrial in origin:

- **Matching upright Ps, atrial rate >160 at rest,** *or*
- **No Ps at all; wavy or sawtooth baseline between QRSs present instead,** *or*
- **P waves of ≥ three different shapes,** *or*
- **Premature abnormal P wave (with or without QRS) interrupting another rhythm,** *or*
- **Heart rate ≥130, rhythm regular, P waves not discernible (may be present, but can't be sure)**

Atrial Rhythms Pictorial

Wandering Atrial Pacemaker (WAP)

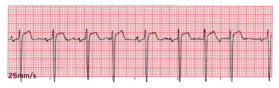

Criteria: Irregular rhythm with at least three different shapes of P waves, mean HR <100. PR interval varies, QRS interval <0.12 secs.

Cause: Hypoxia, medication side effects, vagal stimulation, MI.

Adverse Effects: Usually none.

Treatment: Usually none needed.

Multifocal Atrial Tachycardia (MAT)

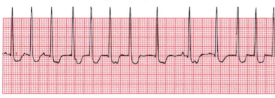

Criteria: Same rhythm as wandering atrial pacemaker, but with a HR >100.

Cause: Chronic lung disease (COPD), heart disease.

Adverse Effects: Signs of decreased cardiac output if HR too fast.

Treatment: Beta-blockers or calcium channel blockers.

Atrial Rhythms Pictorial (cont'd)

PACs

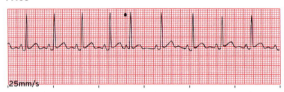

,25mm/s

Criteria: Premature, abnormally shaped P wave followed by a QRS. PACs usually interrupt some sort of sinus rhythm. PR may differ from those on sinus beats, QRS interval <0.12 secs.

Cause: Stimulants, hypoxia, heart disease, early heart failure.

Adverse Effects: Usually none.

Treatment: Remove stimulants. May need digitalis, beta-blockers, calcium channel blockers. May start oxygen.

Nonconducted PAC

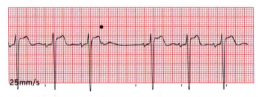

25mm/s

Criteria: Premature, abnormally shaped P wave *not* followed by a QRS. Nonconducted PACs usually interrupt a sinus rhythm of some sort. Results in a pause.

Cause: PAC is so early it can't conduct to the ventricles, which are still refractory.

Adverse Effects: Usually none. Long or frequent pauses can cause signs of decreased cardiac output.

Treatment: Usually none needed.

Atrial Rhythms Pictorial (cont'd)

Paroxysmal Atrial Tachycardia (PAT)

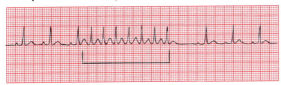

Criteria: This is a burst of three or more PACs that interrupts a sinus rhythm. Atrial tachycardia's HR is 160 to 250,
regular. PR interval differs from sinus PR, QRS interval
<0.12 secs.
Cause: Same as PACs.
Adverse Effects: Signs of decreased cardiac output if HR too
fast for too long.
Treatment: Digitalis, beta-blockers, calcium channel blockers,
sedation, amiodarone, oxygen.

Atrial Flutter (AF)

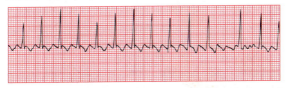

Criteria: Regularly spaced zigzag or sawtooth-shaped
waves between the QRS complexes. No PR interval
because no P waves. QRS interval <0.12 secs.
Cause: Heart disease, pulmonary embolus, valvular heart
disease, lung disease.

Atrial Rhythms Pictorial (cont'd)

Adverse Effects: None at normal HR; signs of decreased cardiac output at higher or lower HRs.

Treatment: Digitalis, beta-blockers, calcium channel blockers, adenosine, electrical cardioversion, carotid sinus massage, oxygen.

Atrial Fibrillation (Afib)

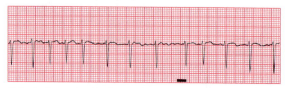

Criteria: Irregular rhythm with wavy or undulating baseline between QRS complexes. There are no P waves, so no PR interval. QRS interval <0.12 secs.

Cause: MI, lung disease, valvular heart disease, hyperthyroidism.

Adverse Effects: Signs of decreased cardiac output; stroke, MI, pulmonary embolus. Blood clots can form in the wiggling atria.

Treatment: If <48 hours duration, goal is to convert rhythm to sinus–give digitalis, calcium channel blockers, beta-blockers, amiodarone, electrical cardioversion. If >48 hours, start anticoagulation and wait 2–3 weeks, then try to convert rhythm to sinus. Start oxygen.

Atrial Rhythms Pictorial (cont'd)

Supraventricular Tachycardia (SVT)

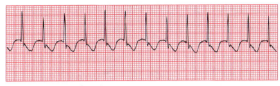

Criteria: Regular rhythm with narrow QRS complex and indistinguishable P waves, HR ≥130. The origin of the rhythm is unclear but is above the ventricle, as evidenced by the QRS interval of <0.12 secs.

Cause: Same as PACs.

Adverse Effects: Signs of decreased cardiac output at higher heart rates.

Treatment: Oxygen, digitalis, adenosine, beta-blockers, calcium channel blockers, electrical cardioversion.

How to Identify Junctional Rhythms

Junctional rhythms are seen less often than sinus or atrial rhythms. Though the inherent rate of the AV junction is 40 to 60, the heart rate may actually go much faster or slower, and can result in symptoms. More normal heart rates are less likely to cause symptoms.

Treatment is aimed at alleviating the cause of the junctional rhythm. More active treatment is not usually necessary unless symptoms develop, at which time the goal is to convert the rhythm back to sinus or to return the heart rate to more normal levels.

Junctional rhythms are very easy to identify. Here are the criteria:

Regular rhythm or premature beat with narrow QRS and one of the following:

- Absent P waves
- Inverted P waves following the QRS
- Inverted P waves with short PR interval preceding the QRS

Junctional Rhythms Pictorial

PJCs

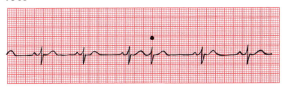

Criteria: Premature beat with inverted or absent P wave interrupting a sinus rhythm of some sort. PR interval <0.12 secs if inverted P precedes the QRS. QRS interval <0.12 secs.
Cause: Stimulants, hypoxia, heart disease.
Adverse Effects: None.
Treatment: Remove the cause.

Junctional Bradycardia (JB)

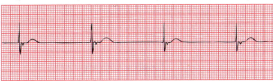

Criteria: Regular rhythm with inverted or absent P waves, HR <40. PR <0.12 secs if inverted P precedes the QRS. QRS interval <0.12 secs.
Cause: Vagal stimulation, hypoxia, sinus node ischemia, heart disease, medications.
Adverse Effects: Signs of decreased cardiac output.
Treatment: Remove the cause. Give atropine, oxygen, transcutaneous pacemaker, epinephrine or dopamine infusion if symptomatic.

Junctional Rhythms Pictorial (cont'd)

Junctional Rhythm (JR)

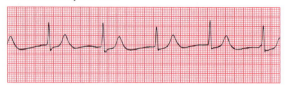

Criteria: Same as junctional bradycardia, except HR 40 to 60.
Cause, adverse effects, treatment: Same as junctional bradycardia.

Accelerated Junctional Rhythm (AJR)

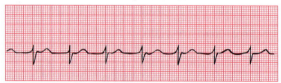

Criteria: Same as junctional rhythm, except HR 60–100.
Cause: Heart disease, stimulant drugs, caffeine.
Adverse Effects: Usually none as HR is normal.
Treatment: Treat the cause.

Junctional Rhythms Pictorial (cont'd)

Junctional Tachycardia (JT)

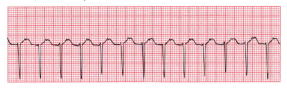

Criteria: Same as AJR, except HR >100. Call this rhythm SVT if P wave not seen.

Cause: Heart disease, stimulants; most often caused by digitalis toxicity.

Adverse Effects: Signs of decreased cardiac output if HR too fast.

Treatment: Oxygen, beta-blockers, calcium channel blockers, electrical cardioversion. Hold digitalis if that's the cause.

How to Identify Ventricular Rhythms

Ventricular rhythms are the most lethal of all rhythms and command great respect from healthcare personnel. They can result from escape (the inherent rate of the ventricle is 20 to 40) or usurpation, and can have a heart rate varying from 0 to over 250 beats per minute. Though some ventricular rhythms can be well tolerated, most will cause symptoms of decreased cardiac output, if not frank cardiac standstill.

Though most ventricular rhythms respond well to medications, some of the very medications used to treat ventricular rhythms can *cause* them in some circumstances. Some ventricular rhythms can only be treated by electric shock to the heart. And others, despite aggressive treatment, are usually lethal.

Ventricular beats have wide, bizarre QRS complexes. Some ventricular rhythms, however, have no QRS complexes at all. If the rhythm or beat in question meets *either* of the following criteria, it is ventricular in origin:

- Wide QRS (>0.12 secs) without preceding P wave, *or*
- No QRS at all (or can't tell if there are QRS complexes) *or*
- Premature, wide QRS beat without preceding P wave, interrupting another rhythm

---

Ventricular Rhythms Pictorial

PVCs

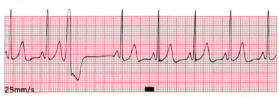

25mm/s

Criteria: Premature wide-QRS beat without preceding P wave, interrupting a sinus rhythm. No P wave so no PR interval, QRS interval >0.12 secs.
Cause: Heart disease, hypokalemia, hypoxia, stimulants, hypomagnesemia.
Adverse Effects: Can progress to ventricular tachycardia or ventricular fibrillation.
Treatment: None if PVCs just occasional. Atropine if PVCs in a slow bradycardia. Amiodarone or lidocaine if frequent PVCs. Otherwise treat the cause.

Agonal Rhythm (Dying Heart)

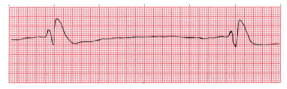

Criteria: Irregular rhythm with QRS interval >0.12 secs and no preceding P wave, HR <20. No PR interval.
Cause: Profound cardiac or other system failure. The patient is dying.

Ventricular Rhythms
Pictorial (cont'd)

Adverse Effects: Profound shock, unconsciousness, death if untreated.
Treatment: CPR, epinephrine, atropine, oxygen.

Idioventricular Rhythm (IVR)

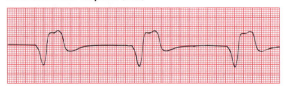

Criteria: Same as agonal rhythm except HR 20 to 40 and rhythm regular.
Cause, adverse effects, treatment: Same as agonal rhythm at slower end of HR. May be tolerated at faster HR.

Accelerated Idioventricular Rhythm (AIVR)

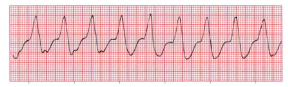

Criteria: Same as IVR except HR 40 to 100.
Cause: Same as for PVCs.
Adverse Effects: Usually none as HR normal.
Treatment: Atropine if HR slow and symptoms. Oxygen.

Ventricular Rhythms Pictorial (cont'd)

Ventricular Tachycardia (V-tach)

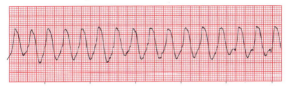

Criteria: Same as AIVR except HR >100.
Cause: Same as for PVCs.
Adverse Effects: Short runs can be tolerated, longer runs can cause cardiovascular collapse, unconsciousness, death if untreated.
Treatment: Defibrillate and start CPR if pulseless. Amiodarone or lidocaine if stable. Treat the cause.

Torsades de Pointes

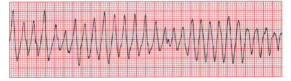

Criteria: Wide QRS without preceding P wave. QRS complexes rotate around an axis, pointing up and down, HR >200. Torsades is recognized more by its characteristic oscillating pattern than by other criteria.
Cause: Same as V-tach. Can also be caused by antiarrhythmic medications such as quinidine, amiodarone, procainamide.

Ventricular Rhythms
Pictorial (cont'd)

Adverse Effects: Short runs can be tolerated, longer runs can cause unconsciousness, shock, death if untreated.

Treatment: Magnesium, electrical cardioversion, or defibrillation. Oxygen.

Ventricular Fibrillation (V-fib)

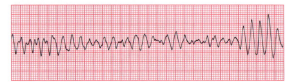

Criteria: No QRS complexes at all, just a wavy baseline looking like static.

Cause: Same as V-tach plus drowning, drug overdoses, accidental electric shock.

Adverse Effects: Pulselessness, death if untreated.

Treatment: Immediate defibrillation, CPR, epinephrine, amiodarone, oxygen, lidocaine.

Ventricular Rhythms Pictorial (cont'd)

Asystole

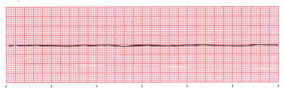

Criteria: No Ps or QRS complexes, flat line only.
Cause: Profound hypoxia or other body system failure. The patient is dying.
Adverse Effects: Pulselessness, death if untreated.
Treatment: CPR, epinephrine, atropine, oxygen. Consider termination of resuscitation.

P Wave Asystole

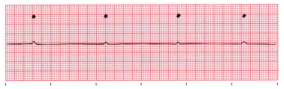

Criteria: No QRS complexes–P waves only.
Cause, adverse effects, treatment: Same as asystole.

How to Identify AV Blocks

In AV blocks, the underlying rhythm is sinus. The impulse is born in the sinus node and heads down the conduction pathway as usual. Thus the P waves are normal sinus P waves. Further down the conduction pathway, however, there is a roadblock that can result in either a delay or an interruption in transmission of sinus impulses to the ventricle. Heart rates can be normal or very slow, and symptoms may or may not be present. Treatment is aimed at increasing the heart rate and improving AV conduction.

There are two possible criteria for AV blocks:

- **PR interval prolonged (>0.20 secs) in some kind of sinus rhythm,** *or*

- **Some Ps not followed by a QRS; P-P interval regular**

AV Blocks Pictorial

First-Degree AV Block

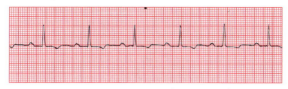

Criteria: Prolonged PR interval (>0.20 secs) in a sinus rhythm of some sort, QRS interval <0.12 secs.
Cause: AV node ischemia, digitalis toxicity, medications.
Adverse Effects: None.
Treatment: Treat the cause.

Mobitz I Second-Degree AV Block (Wenckebach)

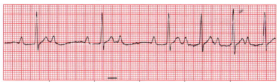

Criteria: P-P regular, PR interval varies, R-R interval varies. PR intervals gradually prolong until one P is not followed by a QRS. QRS interval <0.12 secs.
Cause: MI, digitalis toxicity, medications.
Adverse Effects: Usually none as HR is normal.
Treatment: Usually none needed. Atropine, transcutaneous pacing if symptoms.

AV Blocks Pictorial (cont'd)

Mobitz II Second-Degree AV Block

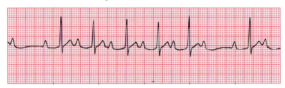

Criteria: P-P regular, PR interval constant on the conducted beats, some Ps not followed by a QRS. QRS interval <0.12 secs if block is at AV node, ≥0.12 secs if block at bundle branches.
Cause: MI, conduction system lesion, hypoxia, medications.
Adverse Effects: Signs of decreased cardiac output at slower HR.
Treatment: Pacemaker, atropine, epinephrine or dopamine infusion, oxygen.

2:1 AV Block

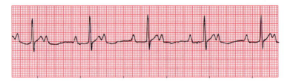

Criteria: P-P regular, R-R regular, PR interval constant. Only every other P wave is followed by a QRS.
Causes, adverse effects, treatment: Same as Wenckebach or Mobitz II.

AV Blocks Pictorial (cont'd)

Third-Degree AV Block (Complete Heart Block)

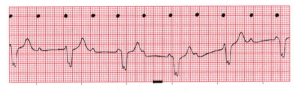

Criteria: P-P regular, R-R regular, PR intervals vary. Atrial rate is faster than ventricular rate. Some Ps are not followed by a QRS. There is complete AV dissociation. None of the P waves is associated with the QRS complexes, even though at times there may appear to be a relationship. QRS interval <0.12 secs if block at AV node, >0.12 secs if block at bundle branches. Junctional or ventricular escape beats provide the QRS complex.

Cause: MI, conduction system lesion, hypoxia, medications.

Adverse Effects: Signs of decreased cardiac output.

Treatment: Pacemaker, atropine, epinephrine or dopamine infusion, oxygen.

How to Identify Pacemaker Rhythms

Pacemaker rhythms are generated by an electrical stimulus from an attached or implanted pacemaker generator. A three-letter code identifies the type of pacemaker in use. The first letter refers to the chamber paced, the second is the chamber sensed, and the third is the response to sensed events. Pacing can involve the atrium, the ventricle, or both. VVI pacemakers pace only the ventricle. DDD pacemakers pace atrium and ventricle.

Here are the criteria for pacemaker rhythms:

- All paced rhythms will have a pacemaker spike, a thin vertical line, immediately preceding paced beats.

- If the ventricle is paced, the resultant QRS will be wide, resembling ventricular beats.

Pacemaker Rhythms Pictorial

Ventricular Pacing (VVI)

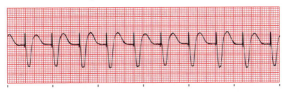

Criteria: Pacemaker spike before each wide QRS complex, QRS interval >0.12 secs.

Dual Chamber Pacing (DDD)

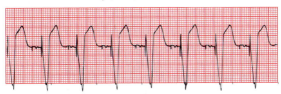

Criteria: Spike before the P wave and before the wide QRS.

How to Identify Pacemaker Malfunctions

There are three types of pacemaker malfunctions:

1. **Failure to fire.** The pacemaker has failed to generate an impulse, perhaps because its battery is dead or the connecting wires are disrupted. Failure to fire is recognized by the absence of pacemaker spikes where they should have been.

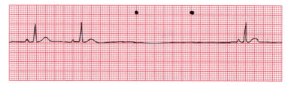

2. **Loss of capture.** The pacemaker has fired–there are pacemaker spikes–but there is no P wave or QRS following that spike. The pacemaker is not generating enough "juice" to cause the chamber to respond to the pacemaker's signal. Turning up the pacemaker's voltage often corrects this problem.

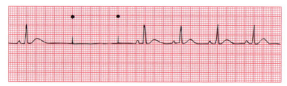

How to Identify Pacemaker Malfunctions (cont'd)

3. **Undersensing.** The pacemaker does not sense ("see") the patient's own intrinsic beats, so it fires as if those beats weren't there. This results in paced beats or pacemaker spikes inside QRS complexes, in ST segments, or in other places too close to the intrinsic beats.

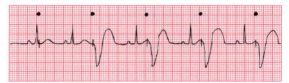

12-Lead EKG Interpretation

How to Place Leads for a Standard 12-Lead EKG

Limb leads are on each arm and leg. Limb leads are leads I, II, III, aVR, aVL, and aVF. **Precordial** (**chest**) **leads** are located on the left chest. They are named V_1, V_2, V_3, V_4, V_5, and V_6.

Location of the Precordial Leads

V_1 Fourth intercostal space, right sternal border (abbreviated 4th ICS, RSB)

V_2 Fourth intercostal space, left sternal border (4th ICS, LSB)

V_3 Between V_2 and V_4

V_4 Fifth intercostal space, left midclavicular line (5th ICS, MCL)

V_5 Fifth intercostal space, left anterior axillary line (5th ICS, AAL)

V_6 Fifth intercostal space, left midaxillary line (5th ICS, MAL)

Intercostal spaces are the spaces between the ribs. The fourth intercostal space is the space *below* the fourth rib; the fifth intercostal space is below the fifth rib, and so on. The **midclavicular line** is a line down from the middle of the clavicle (collarbone). The **anterior axillary line** is a line down from the front of the axilla (armpit). The **midaxillary line** is down from the middle of the axilla.

How to Place Leads for a Standard 12-Lead EKG (cont'd)

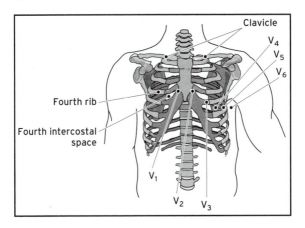

How to Interpret 12-Lead EKGs (Criteria)

Here's a breakdown of what you need to look for on every 12-lead EKG:

The Basics	Rhythm, rate, intervals (PR, QRS, QT)
Axis Quadrant	Normal, LAD, RAD, or indeterminate?
Bundle branch block/Hemiblock	RBBB = RSR′ in V_1, QRS ≥ 0.12 secs LBBB = QS or RS in V_1, QRS ≥ 0.12 secs LAHB = Small Q in I, small R in III, left axis deviation LPHB = Small R in I, small Q in III, right axis deviation
Hypertrophy	RVH = R ≥ S in V_1, inverted T, right axis deviation LVH = S in V_1 + R in V_5 or V_6 ≥ 35
Myocardial Infarction/ Ischemia	Anterior MI = ST elevation and/or significant Q in V_2 to V_4 Inferior MI = ST elevation and/or significant Q in II, III, aVF Lateral MI = ST elevation and/or significant Q in I, aVL, V_5 to V_6 Anteroseptal MI = ST elevation and/or significant Q in V_1 plus any anterior lead(s) Extensive anterior (extensive anterior-lateral) MI = ST elevation and/or significant Q in I, aVL, V_1 to V_6 Posterior MI = Large R + upright T in V_1 to V_2; may also have ST depression NSTEMI = Widespread ST depression and T wave inversion in many leads Ischemia = Inverted T waves in any lead, as long as not BBB-related
Miscellaneous Effects	Digitalis effect = Sagging ST segments, prolonged PR interval Hyperkalemia = Tall, pointy, narrow T waves Severe hyperkalemia = Wide QRS complex Hypokalemia = Prominent U waves, flattened T waves Hypercalcemia = Shortened ST segment causing short QT interval Hypocalcemia = Prolonged ST segment causing prolonged QT interval

How to Interpret 12-Lead EKGs (Checklist)

Use this checklist to document your findings on 12-lead EKGs.

The Basics
• Rhythm _____

• Rate _____

• Intervals   PR _____ QRS _____ QT _____

Axis
Circle correct choice:

Normal   LAD   RAD   Indeterminate

Bundle Branch Blocks/Hemiblocks
Circle if present:

RBBB   LBBB   LAHB   LPHB

Hypertrophy
Circle if present:

RVH   LVH

Infarction/Ischemia
Circle if present:

Infarction   Ischemia

Which wall(s) of the heart? _____.

How to Interpret 12-Lead EKGs (Checklist) (cont'd)

Miscellaneous Effects

Circle if present:

Digitalis effect

Hyperkalemia

Severe hyperkalemia

Hypokalemia

Hypercalcemia

Hypocalcemia

How to Determine the Axis Quadrant

Look at the QRS in leads I and aVF to determine the axis quadrant. Because lead I joins right arm and left arm, it tells us whether the heart's current is traveling to the right or left. AVF's positive pole is on the leg, so it tells us if the heart's current is traveling upward or downward.

If the QRS complexes in leads I and aVF are both positive, the axis is in the normal quadrant. If leads I and aVF are both negative, it's an indeterminate axis. If lead I is positive and aVF is negative, it's left axis deviation (LAD). If lead I is negative and aVF is positive, it's right axis deviation (RAD).

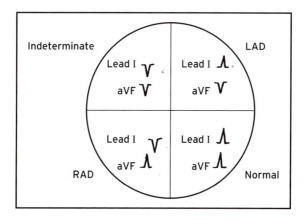

How to Identify Bundle Branch Blocks/Hemiblocks (Criteria)

Criteria for Bundle Branch Blocks

	QRS configuration in V_1	QRS configuration in V_6	QRS interval	T wave
RBBB	RSR'	QRS (wide terminal S)	≥0.12 secs	Opposite the terminal QRS
LBBB	QS or RS	Monophasic R	≥0.12 secs	Opposite the terminal QRS

Criteria for Hemiblocks

	Lead I	Lead III	QRS interval	Axis
LAHB	Small Q, taller R	Sm R, deeper S	<0.12 secs	Left axis deviation
LPHB	Small R, deeper S	Sm Q, taller R	<0.12 secs	Right axis deviation

How to Identify Bundle Branch Blocks/Hemiblocks (Algorithm)

Use this algorithm to determine if there is a BBB or hemiblock, or both, on the EKG. Just answer the questions and follow the arrows to the answer.

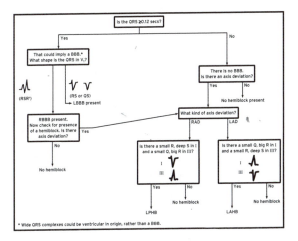

How to Recognize a STEMI (ST Elevation MI) As It Evolves

Timeline	Age of MI	EKG Change	Implication
Immediately before the actual MI starts		T wave inversion	Cardiac tissue is ischemic, as evidenced by the newly inverted T waves.
Within hours after the MI's start	Acute	Marked ST elevation + upright T wave	Acute MI has begun, starting with myocardial injury.
Hours later	Acute	Significant Q + ST Elevation + upright T	Some of the injured myocardial tissue has died, while other tissue remains injured.
Hours to a day or two later	Acute	Significant Q + less ST elevation + marked T inversion	Infarction is almost complete. Some injury and ischemia persist at the infarct edges.
Days to weeks later (in some cases this stage may last up to a year)	Age indeterminate	Significant Q + T wave inversion	Infarction is complete. Though there is no more ischemic tissue (it has either recovered or died), the T wave inversion persists.
Weeks, months, years later	Old	Significant Q only	The significant Q wave persists, signifying permanent tissue death.

How to Determine the Age of an MI

When an EKG is interpreted, the interpreter does not necessarily know the patient's clinical status and therefore must base determination of the MI's age on the indicative changes that are present on the EKG.

The age of an MI is determined as follows:

- An MI that has ST segment elevation is **acute** (one to two days old or less).

- An MI with significant Q waves, baseline (or almost back to baseline) ST segments, and inverted T waves is of **age indeterminate** (several days old, up to a year in some cases). Some authorities call this a **recent MI.**

- The MI with significant Q waves, baseline ST segments, and upright T waves is **old** (weeks to years old).

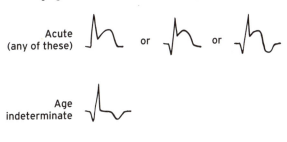

Acute
(any of these)   or   or

Age
indeterminate

Old

How to Identify MI Location (Infarction Squares)

Each lead square is labeled with the wall of the heart at which it looks. When you analyze an EKG, note which leads have ST elevation and/or significant Q waves. Then use the infarction squares to determine the type of infarction. For example, if there were ST elevation in leads II, III, aVF, and V_5 and V_6, you would note that the MI involves inferior and lateral leads. The MI would be inferior-lateral.

I	aVR	V_1	V_4
Lateral	Ignore this lead when looking for MIs	Septal (posterior if mirror image)	Anterior
II	aVL	V_2	V_5
Inferior	Lateral	Anterior (posterior if mirror image)	Lateral
III	aVF	V_3	V_6
Inferior	Inferior	Anterior	Lateral

How to Identify MI Location (Criteria)

Location of MI	EKG Changes	Coronary Artery
Anterior	Indicative changes in V_2 to V_4 Reciprocal changes in II, III, aVF	Left anterior descending (LAD)
Inferior	Indicative changes in II, III, aVF Reciprocal changes in I, aVL, and V leads	Right coronary artery (RCA)
Lateral	Indicative changes in I, aVL, V_5 to V_6 May see reciprocal changes in II, III, aVF	Circumflex
Posterior	No indicative changes, as no leads look directly at posterior wall Diagnosed by reciprocal changes in V_1 and V_2 (large R wave, upright T wave, and possibly ST depression), seen as a mirror image of an anterior MI.	RCA or circumflex
Extensive anterior (sometimes called *extensive anterior-lateral*)	Indicative changes in I, aVL, V_1 to V_6 Reciprocal changes in II, III, aVF	LAD or left main
Anteroseptal	Indicative changes in V_1 plus any anterior lead(s) Usually no reciprocal changes	LAD

Anterior MI Pictorial

An anterior MI damages the front (anterior) wall of the left ventricle. It is a large MI. Look for EKG changes in leads V_2 to V_4.

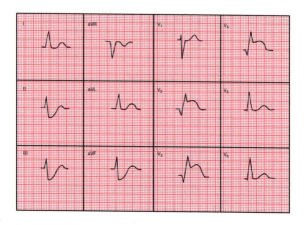

This is an **acute anterior MI,** as evidenced by the ST elevation in V_2 to V_4. Also note the reciprocal ST depression in leads II, III, and aVF.

If this MI were **age indeterminate,** it would have more normal ST segments, significant Q waves, and T wave inversions in V_2 to V_4.

If this MI were **old,** it would have only the significant Q wave remaining. The ST segment would be back at baseline and the T wave would be upright.

Inferior MI Pictorial

An inferior MI damages the bottom (inferior) wall of the left ventricle. Look for EKG changes in leads II, III, and aVF.

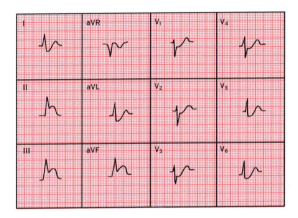

This is an **acute inferior MI.** Note the ST elevation in leads II, III, and aVF. Note also the reciprocal ST segment depression in leads I, aVL, and V_1 to V_6.

The **age indeterminate inferior MI** would have more normal ST segments along with significant Q waves and inverted T waves in leads II, III, and aVF.

The **old inferior MI** would have only significant Q waves in II, III, and aVF. The ST segments would be at baseline and T waves would be upright.

Lateral MI Pictorial

Lateral wall MIs damage the left side wall (lateral wall) of
the left ventricle. Look for EKG changes in leads I, aVL,
and V_5 to V_6.

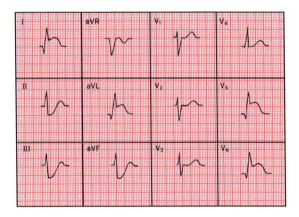

This is an **acute lateral wall MI,** as evidenced by the
ST elevation in leads I, aVL, and V_5 to V_6. Note also the
reciprocal ST depression in leads II, III, and aVF.

If this were an **age indeterminate lateral MI,** there
would be more normal ST segments along with significant
Q waves and inverted T waves in I, aVL, and V_5 to V_6.

An **old lateral wall MI** would have baseline ST
segments, significant Q waves, and upright T waves in I,
aVL, and V_5 to V_6.

Posterior MI Pictorial

Posterior MIs damage the back (posterior) wall of the left ventricle. Because we don't routinely put EKG leads on the back, we are not able to see a posterior MI in the same way as other MIs. With other MIs, we look directly at the damaged area by way of the leads placed directly over that area. For posterior MIs, we look through the front of the heart to see the back. It's rather like looking through the front of a cola bottle to see the very back. What we'd see on the front is the mirror image of what's on the back. For other types of MIs, we look for ST elevation, Q waves, and inverted T waves. For posterior MIs, we look for big R waves (the mirror image of a Q wave), ST depression (the mirror image of ST elevation), and upright T waves (the mirror image of inverted T waves). Look for these EKG changes in V_1 and V_2.

Posterior MIs almost always accompany an inferior MI, so always look in leads II, III, and aVF for the inferior MI.

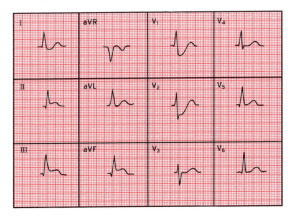

Posterior MI Pictorial (cont'd)

This is an **acute posterior wall MI.** Note the tall R wave in V_1 to V_2 along with ST segment depression and an upright T wave. Note also that there is an acute inferior MI as well.

An **age indeterminate posterior MI** would have more normal ST segments, a tall R wave, and an upright T wave.

The **old posterior MI** would have only the tall R wave remaining. The ST segments would be at baseline and the T wave would be inverted.

Extensive Anterior MI Pictorial (Also Called Extensive Anterior-Lateral MI)

An extensive anterior MI is a huge, often catastrophic, MI. It damages the anterior and lateral walls of the left ventricle. Look for EKG changes in leads I, aVL, and V_1 to V_6.

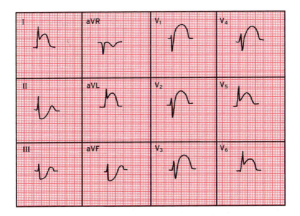

Here we have a huge MI, the **acute extensive anterior MI.** Note the ST elevation in I, aVL, and V_1 to V_6 and the reciprocal ST depression in II, III, and aVF.

The **age indeterminate extensive anterior MI** would have more normal ST segments along with significant Q waves and T wave inversion.

The **old extensive anterior MI** would have baseline ST segments, significant Q waves, and upright T waves in I, aVL, and V_1 to V_6.

Anteroseptal MI Pictorial

An anteroseptal MI is a small MI that damages the septum and part of the anterior wall. Look for EKG changes in V_1 plus any anterior lead(s).

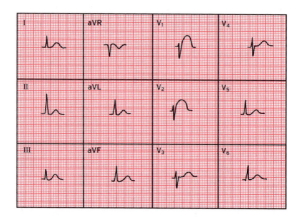

This is an **acute anteroseptal MI.** Note the ST elevation in leads V_1 to V_2.

An **age indeterminate anteroseptal MI** would have more normal ST segments, significant Q waves, and inverted T waves in the involved leads.

The **old anteroseptal MI** would have only significant Q waves remaining in the involved leads. The ST segments would be at baseline and the T waves would be upright.

NSTEMI Pictorial

A NSTEMI is an MI that damages only the innermost layer of myocardium. Look for widespread changes throughout the 12-lead EKG.

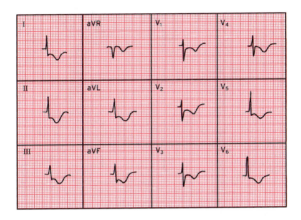

This is an **acute NSTEMI** (non-ST elevation MI). It is characterized by widespread ST depression and T wave inversions. These MIs are diagnosed only in the acute phase, as they do not cause significant Q waves, and their T waves are already inverted.

How to Identify MI Location (Algorithm)

This algorithm is designed to point out the myocardial infarction area. Just answer the questions and follow the arrows.

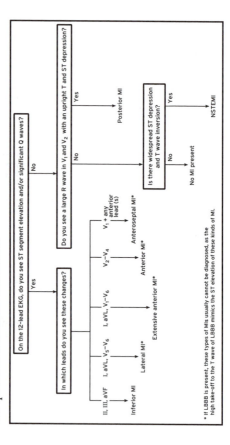

* If LBBB is present, these types of MIs usually cannot be diagnosed, as the high take-off to the T wave of LBBB mimics the ST elevation of these kinds of MI.

How to Place Leads For a Right-Sided EKG

A right-sided EKG is done with the limb leads in their normal places, but with the precordial leads placed on the right side of the chest instead of the left. Right-sided EKGs are used to diagnose right ventricular infarctions.

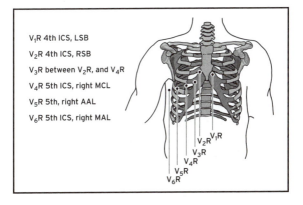

V₁R 4th ICS, LSB

V₂R 4th ICS, RSB

V₃R between V₂R, and V₄R

V₄R 5th ICS, right MCL

V₅R 5th, right AAL

V₆R 5th ICS, right MAL

V₂R V₁R
V₃R
V₄R
V₅R
V₆R

How to Identify Right Ventricular Infarction

Right ventricular infarctions are not as common as MIs that affect the left ventricle. When seen, right ventricular infarctions accompany an inferior wall MI. Right ventricular infarctions are recognized by ST segment elevation in right-sided EKG leads V_3R or V_4R. A standard EKG, which looks at the left ventricle, will not pick up a right ventricular infarction.

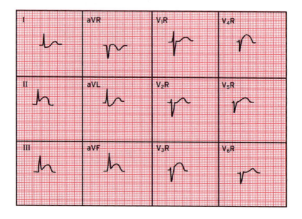

On this right-sided EKG, note the ST elevation in leads V_3R to V_4R. This proves there is an RV infarction. You'll note also that there is ST elevation in leads II, III, and aVF that indicate an inferior MI. Remember, the right-sided EKG leaves the limb leads in their normal place, but moves the precordial leads to the right side of the chest. So the inferior MI will still be obvious on the right-sided EKG.

How to Identify Pericarditis

Pericarditis is an inflammation of the pericardial sac, the sac that surrounds the heart. The myocardial layer just beneath this inflamed pericardium also becomes inflamed, causing temporary EKG changes that can mimic the changes seen with an acute MI. Pericarditis is recognized by widespread concave ST elevation.

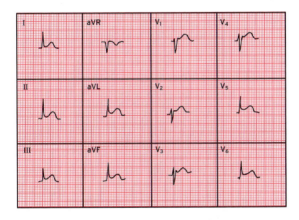

Note the widespread concave ST elevation in leads I, II, III, aVL, aVF, and V_1 to V_6. This is *not* typical of an MI because it is so widespread. Is it possible this is a huge MI instead of pericarditis? Sure. But based on the concave ST elevation scattered across many leads, it's more likely that it's pericarditis. Only by examining the patient would we know for sure.

How to Identify Early Repolarization

Early repolarization is a variation of a normal EKG. Repolarization begins so early in this condition that the T wave appears to start before the QRS has even finished. This makes it look like the ST segment is slightly elevated, mimicking an MI. There is often a "fishhook" at the end of some QRS complexes that gives a hint that there is early repolarization.

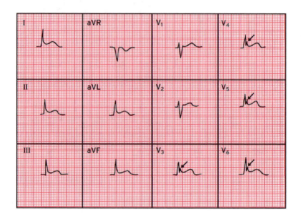

In this EKG, note the mild ST segment elevation in almost all leads and the fishhook in V_3 to V_6 (see arrows). This is typical of early repolarization.

How to Identify Miscellaneous EKG Effects

Effect	EKG Change

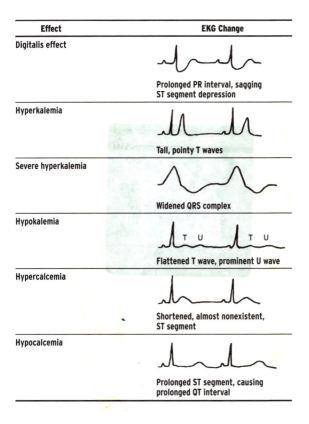

Digitalis effect

Prolonged PR interval, sagging ST segment depression

Hyperkalemia

Tall, pointy T waves

Severe hyperkalemia

Widened QRS complex

Hypokalemia

T U   T U

Flattened T wave, prominent U wave

Hypercalcemia

Shortened, almost nonexistent, ST segment

Hypocalcemia

Prolonged ST segment, causing prolonged QT interval

RC 683.5 E5 E44 2012
Ellis, Karen M.,
EKG in a heartbeat

DATE DUE

Index